TAKE HEART

Jill Howard and Belinda Morieson are both experienced coronary care nurses. Their education programme for people recovering from heart attack or cardiac surgery has been acclaimed Australia-wide. They have both been working in nursing for 30 years.

Jill Howard is currently a Director of Nursing at Monash Medical Centre and was the founding member of the Victorian Cardiac Nurses Association.

Belinda Morieson was a Senior Coronary Care Nurse at Prince Henry's Hospital and is now Secretary of the Australian Nursing Federation (Victorian branch).

Andrea McCance is the Nurse Program Director of Heart and Chest Services at Southern Healthcare Network. Until recently she was the Nurse Unit Manager of Cardiac Care at Monash Medical Centre. She has contributed her wealth of knowledge to this revised edition of *Take Heart*.

TAKE HEART

A Guide to Recovery after a Heart Attack

Revised Edition

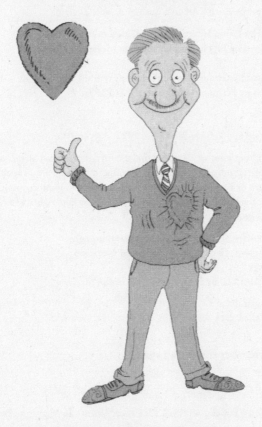

Jill Howard & Belinda Morieson

with Andrea McCance

VIKING

Viking
Penguin Books Australia Ltd
487 Maroondah Highway, PO Box 257
Ringwood, Victoria 3134, Australia
Penguin Books Ltd
Harmondsworth, Middlesex, England
Viking Penguin, A Division of Penguin Books USA Inc.
375 Hudson Street, New York, New York 10014, USA
Penguin Books Canada Limited
10 Alcorn Avenue, Toronto, Ontario, Canada M4V 3B2
Penguin Books (N.Z.) Ltd
Cnr Rosedale and Airborne Roads, Albany, Auckland, New Zealand

First edition published by Prince Henry's Hospital, Melbourne 1979
Revised edition published by Jill Howard and Belinda Morieson 1985
Reprinted 1986
Second edition published by Greenhouse Publications Pty Ltd 1989
Third edition published by Penguin Books Australia Ltd 1997

10 9 8 7 6 5 4 3 2 1

Typeset in 8/11 pt Sabon by Midland Typesetters, Maryborough
Cartoons by Warren Brown, George Hadden and Ben Morieson
Diagrams by Alan Laver
Printed and bound in Australia by Australian Print Group, Maryborough

National Library of Australia
Cataloguing-in-Publication data

Howard, Jill.
Take heart: a guide to recovery after a heart attack.

Rev. ed.
ISBN 0 670 87109 5.

1. Myocardial infarction – Popular works. I. McCance, Andrea. II. Morieson, Belinda.
III. Title.

616.123703

Foreword

Take Heart, first published in 1979, was based on an innovative patient education programme developed by the staff of the Prince Henry's Hospital coronary care unit, then regarded as one of the best and most progressive units in the world. The aim of the book was to help heart attack patients obtain a healthier and more enjoyable life than before the event. The authors, Jill Howard and Belinda Morieson, were experienced coronary care nurses. Using humorous diagrams and simple direct language free of unnecessary medical jargon, they were able to communicate with their target audience of patients and their families in a way that other medical texts could not.

The book was an instant success. It rapidly became a standard text for coronary care units throughout Australia and has been revised and reprinted many times. Thousands of patients and their families have benefited from the sound practical advice contained within the book.

In 1989 Prince Henry's Hospital closed at its St Kilda Road, Melbourne site. Fortunately the expertise, enthusiasm and innovation so characteristic of the coronary care unit has not been lost. Prince Henry's coronary care unit combined with the unit already at Monash Medical Centre to form the current Monash Medical Centre cardiac care unit.

Jill Howard and Belinda Morieson have gone on to new challenges and the task of updating and rewriting the new edition has fallen on the capable shoulders of Andrea McCance and her nursing colleagues. They are to be congratulated for their efforts. The unique blend of humour and optimism is retained. The language remains simple and concise. The diagrams are explicit, humorous and to the point. Consistent with modern practice, greater emphasis has been placed on interventional cardiology, and new developments such as coronary stents are discussed and explained in terms that are easy to understand. At no stage is technology allowed to dominate. Technology is merely an aid to recovery – a process that requires the integrated total approach so well described in this book.

Take Heart will continue to stimulate, educate and delight patients in coronary care units throughout this country.

Associate Professor Richard Harper
Director of Cardiology,
Monash Medical Centre

Contents

Acknowledgements

Take Heart has been revised and reprinted several times since it was first published in 1979 and is now widely used in hospitals throughout Australia.

Valuable contributors to the first edition were Meredith Spencer (coronary care nurse), Helga Erlanger (social worker), David Rollo (cardiologist) and Warren Brown (artist).

We wish to thank Prince Henry's Hospital (PHH) coronary care nursing staff, Dr Andris Saltups, PHH management, and PHH patients (plus their friends and relatives) for invaluable help and support.

Special thanks to Andrea McCance and her coronary care nursing colleagues at Monash Medical Centre for kindly agreeing to update the 1997 edition of *Take Heart*.

INTRODUCTION

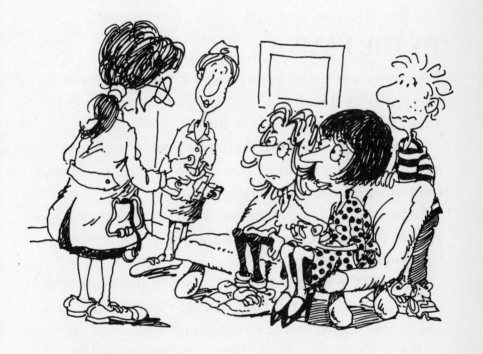

This book answers your questions about heart attack and gives advice on speedy recovery. It includes sections on medications, angina, blood pressure, smoking, diet, exercise and coronary investigative and interventional procedures.

We have intentionally kept language simple and free from 'medical jargon' but have often included medical terms as well as the common terms so that you will know what the medical terms refer to. Large print, drawings, humorous cartoons and diagrams make for easy reading.

We suggest that you read through this book more than once and keep it handy as a ready reference.

TO THE FAMILY

This event was undoubtedly a shock for you too – it was probably unexpected and ill-timed. You will feel anxious and uncertain of the future.

We want to assure you that most people who have had a heart attack will recover and return to a normal, sometimes healthier lifestyle.

Some of the advice about smoking, diets and exercises applies to you too. Take this opportunity to improve your own lifestyle.

We hope the information contained in this book will help you to understand your relative's heart attack and the various aspects of recovery. Should you need any further support or advice do not hesitate to ask the coronary care staff at your hospital. They will be willing to assist you.

YOUR HEART ATTACK

PAIN!

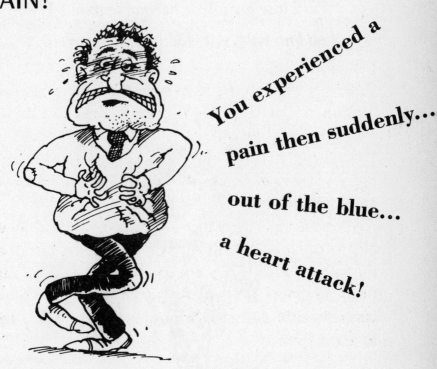

You experienced a pain then suddenly... out of the blue... a heart attack!

Maybe the pain was severe but that doesn't necessarily mean you had a 'severe' heart attack.

CONFUSION

Illness is often considered the unfortunate experience of others. Now that it has happened to you, you may find yourself thinking things like:

'I don't believe it; it was only indigestion.'

'I've been well all my life. How could I have had a heart attack?'

'The pain was terrible. Will it return?'

'Will I lose my job or be unable to work?'

'I had no pain, only tightness in my chest.'

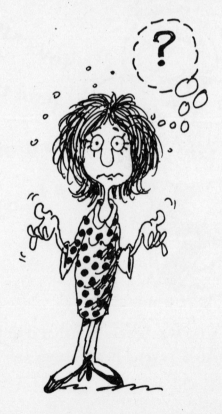

After a heart attack some people imagine they may become an invalid and be unable to do any physical work. This may also be associated with feelings of weakness, self-doubt or fear of dying.

These feelings are temporary. This book will tell you about the various stages of recovery.

MEDICAL TERMINOLOGY

The common medical term for 'heart attack' is 'myocardial infarction'. It is also called:

- a coronary
- a coronary thrombosis
- a coronary occlusion.

These terms all mean 'heart attack'.

HOW IS HEART ATTACK DIAGNOSED?

Symptoms

Common symptoms include:

- a heavy, tight or crushing pain or discomfort in the centre of the chest. This may spread to the arms, neck, jaw or back

- nausea
- vomiting
- sweating
- shortness of breath
- dizziness
- occasionally loss of consciousness.

A heart attack rarely occurs without any of the above symptoms.

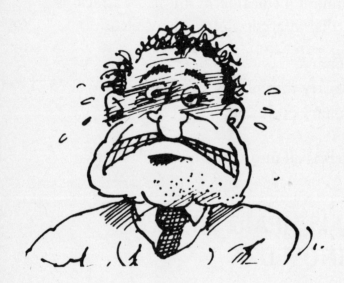

Physical Examination

A physical examination will involve checking:

- blood pressure
- heart sounds
- chest sounds.

Blood Tests

The heart muscle contains substances called 'enzymes' – injury releases these into the bloodstream. Laboratory tests of your blood will detect enzyme release.

Electrocardiograph (ECG)

Electrocardiographs may show some changes indicating that a heart attack has occurred by recording the electrical impulses travelling through the heart muscle.

Echocardiograph

An echocardiograph is an ultrasound examination of the heart which detects abnormalities by recording the movement of the heart valves and chamber walls.

Chest X-ray

A chest X-ray will outline the size of the heart and indicate if there is fluid on the lungs caused by injury to the heart.

HOW YOUR HEART WORKS

Your heart is a muscular pump. This pump requires oxygen to work.

The right side of the heart receives unoxygenated blood from the body and pumps it through the lungs via the pulmonary artery. Carbon dioxide and other waste products are breathed out via the pulmonary artery and oxygen is picked up by the blood.

The left side of the heart receives the blood full of oxygen from the lungs and pumps it out of the aorta (main artery) to the body.

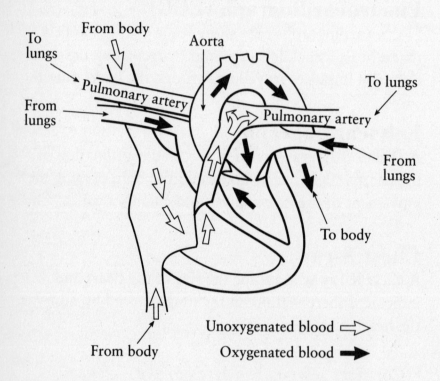

NORMAL CORONARY ARTERIES

Blood vessels called 'coronary arteries' supply oxygen to your heart muscle.

Three main coronary arteries lie on the surface of the heart and divide into smaller branches so that every portion of the heart is supplied with oxygen.

These main coronary arteries are called the anterior, right and circumflex arteries. They originate from the aorta – the body's main artery.

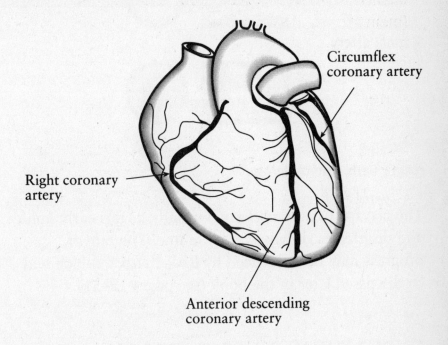

Circumflex coronary artery

Right coronary artery

Anterior descending coronary artery

ATHEROSCLEROSIS

Coronary heart disease develops when arteries supplying blood to the heart muscle become narrowed or obstructed and a part of the heart muscle does not receive enough oxygen.

Atherosclerosis is the build-up over many years of fatty and other materials on the inner lining of an artery causing thickening, narrowing and reduction of blood flow.

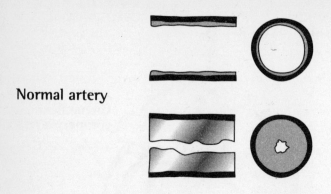

Normal artery

Artery with atherosclerosis

The process of atherosclerosis usually begins early in life and progresses slowly over a lifetime. The rate of progress may be influenced by Risk Factors, which will be discussed later in the book (see pages 19–31).

EXPLAINING HEART ATTACK

Your heart attack occurred when adequate blood flow ceased temporarily in an artery narrowed by atherosclerosis. Because of this inadequate blood flow a small portion of heart muscle was injured and caused the pain you felt.

Blood flow can also be stopped by a blood clot or sudden spasm of a coronary artery.

The damage caused to the heart muscle when the blood flow temporarily stops is called a 'heart attack'.

THE HEALING PROCESS

As with other injuries to the body the injured part of the heart will heal but requires time to do so.

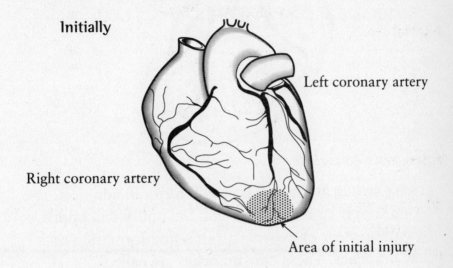

Initially

Left coronary artery

Right coronary artery

Area of initial injury

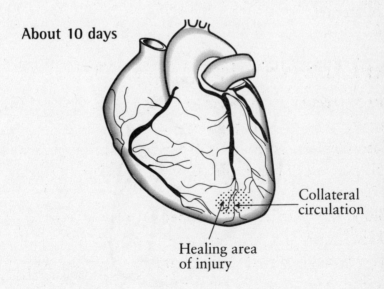

About 10 days

Collateral circulation

Healing area of injury

11

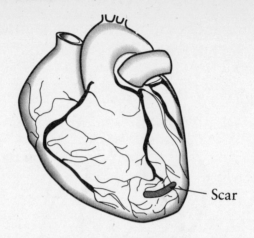

Scar

A very strong and tough scar will form. In addition, blood supply to the area around the injury will improve by enlargement of existing arteries and formation of new branches. These new branches are called 'collaterals'.

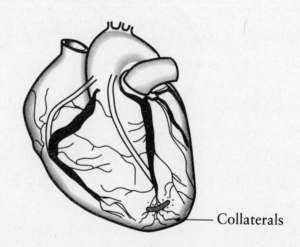

Collaterals

HOSPITAL

THE CORONARY CARE UNIT

Your admission to hospital was probably unexpected; you may have had a fast and disturbing trip and been suddenly confronted with a number of unfamiliar faces and strange pieces of equipment.

When you arrived in the Coronary Care Unit it was our aim to:

- relieve your pain
- establish the correct diagnosis
- observe you closely in order to treat or prevent complications
- administer thrombolytic therapy. The medications Streptokinase or TPA if given within 4 to 24 hours of the onset of pain may dissolve the blood clot blocking the coronary artery, and may potentially reduce the damage to heart muscle
- administer intravenous Heparin and intravenous GTN for 24 to 48 hours. The Heparin helps thin the blood

(so that another clot can't form) while the GTN attempts to keep coronary arteries open.

Monitoring

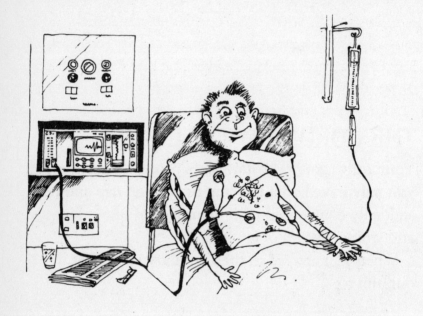

The Coronary Care Unit is a highly specialised area of the hospital. Here specially trained nurses and doctors use electronic equipment to recognise and treat promptly the early signs of complications which can occur after a heart attack.

'Complications' do not necessarily include the onset of a more severe attack or an unduly prolonged recovery. Most complications are of short duration and leave no after effects.

Irregular heart rhythm may occur 24 hours after a

heart attack. Doctors and nurses will detect this on the heart monitor and treat if necessary.

Excess fluid on the lungs could cause shortness of breath. This can be treated with medication which will increase the amount of urine passed.

Pericarditis may occur after a heart attack but generally disappears after a few days. Pericarditis is a short-term problem caused by inflammation of the 'pericardium' (the sac that encloses the heart). The pain may be severe and increase with respiration.

Bed Rest and Length of Stay

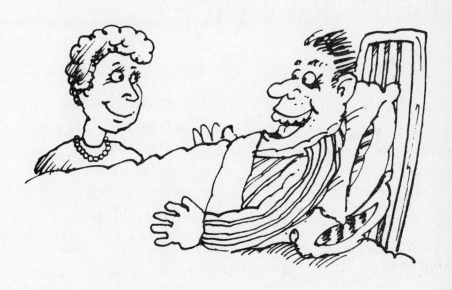

You will stay in the Coronary Care Unit until you are well enough to leave. This is usually 1 to 2 days.

Your initial rest in bed is necessary to start the healing process; however, you are allowed to do most things for yourself from the first day. We try to minimise loss of fitness after your heart attack by keeping you in bed for the shortest possible time.

It has been estimated that for every 24 hours spent in bed we lose 5% of our muscle strength. Most people know that a broken arm kept in plaster for several weeks becomes frail and weak, and requires gradual building up. This same 'deconditioning' process is the main reason you feel weak, easily tired, and sometimes 'woozy' in the head as you begin to move about again.

THE GENERAL WARD

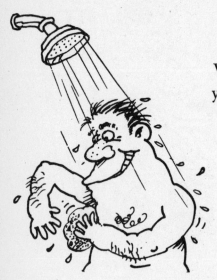

When you are well enough you will be transferred to the General Ward. You may experience some temporary psychological reactions at this time.

Some patients feel insecure after leaving the intensive supervision of a Coronary Care Unit for the General Ward where they are treated like any other convalescing patient. Consider it a promotion – one step closer to home.

Your stay in the General Ward would usually be 3 to 5 days.

While you are in the General Ward the doctors and nurses will advise you to gradually increase your walking distance each day until you are ready to leave the hospital.

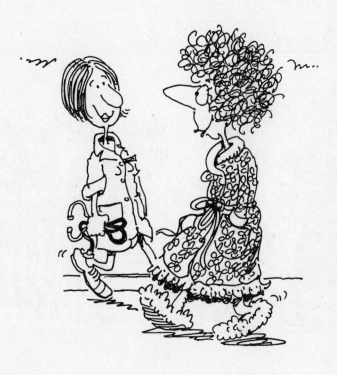

THE SOCIAL WORKER

After a heart attack there are often problems associated with the sudden and unplanned interruption of an accustomed lifestyle.

To ensure that you have as speedy a recovery as possible it is very important to anticipate any areas of concern and anxiety. These may include work, financial or home responsibilities.

If you are not covered by sick pay or are without an income during your illness you may be eligible for sickness benefits.

The social worker involves the whole family to see that no problems are overlooked.

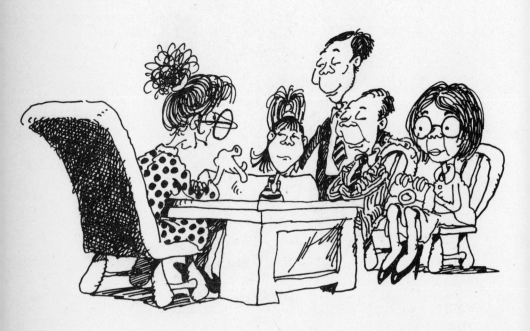

WHY ME?

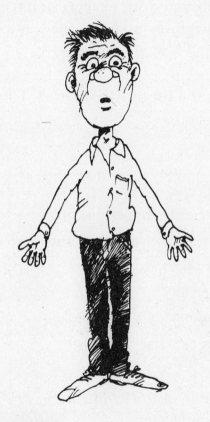

RISK FACTORS

The fundamental cause of heart attack is still uncertain. However, it is known that a number of factors may hasten the narrowing of coronary arteries, thereby increasing the risk of a heart attack. These are called 'Risk Factors'.

Risk Factors are those bodily characteristics and habits that tend to increase your chances of having a heart attack.

Research has shown that the more Risk Factors you have, the greater are your chances of having a heart attack. It is therefore important for you to learn about Risk Factors and how to reduce them.

The following is a list of Risk Factors. How many of these apply to you?

	Yes	No
Smoking		
High blood pressure (hypertension)		
High blood levels of cholesterol and other blood fats		
Overweight (obesity)		
Stress and tension		
Lack of proper exercise		
Diabetes		
Heredity (a family history of heart attack in middle age)		
Menopause		
Being male		
Over 50 years old		

The rest of this chapter provides an explanation of each Risk Factor. Take extra notice of any Risk Factors that apply to you.

SMOKING

Smoking has been identified as a Risk Factor because it:

- constricts your coronary arteries. Remember they may already be narrowed with atherosclerosis
- elevates your blood pressure
- causes abnormalities of your heart rhythm.

Giving up smoking is the most important step in preventing another heart attack but giving up smoking may not be easy!

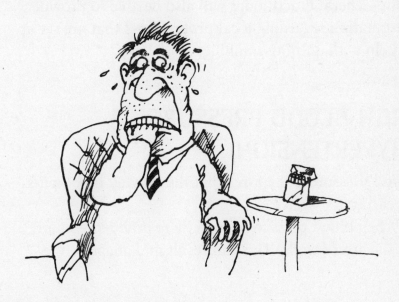

Help Is Available

Discuss it with your doctor or rehabilitation staff. Don't drift back into smoking thinking 'just a few a day won't make any difference'.

Don't switch to a pipe or cigars without discussing it with your doctor – these may not be any safer for you.

There are anti-smoking courses run by:

• Quit Program
• Anti Cancer Council.

Or you may like to consider:

• hypnotherapy
• acupuncture
• nicotine patches or nicotine chewing gum.

Your General Practitioner will also be able to provide information regarding local programmes that are set up to help with quitting smoking.

HIGH BLOOD PRESSURE (HYPERTENSION)

Blood pressure is the force that the moving blood puts on the artery walls.

When blood pressure is high there is added pressure on the artery walls. This can result in damage to the artery which attracts cholesterol and other material to form fatty plaques (atherosclerosis).

Many Australians have high blood pressure yet are unaware of it.

Following your heart attack you should have regular check-ups – at least twice during the first year after the attack.

Treatment for high blood pressure may include:

- weight reduction
- salt restriction
- exercise as prescribed by your doctor
- giving up smoking
- taking prescribed medications.

HIGH BLOOD CHOLESTEROL (AND OTHER BLOOD FATS)

Cholesterol is produced by our bodies and is also found in many of the foods we eat. It is a normal constituent of blood but when we eat more fat than we need (in particular saturated fat), excess cholesterol and other fats may be deposited in the arteries.

The higher the blood cholesterol, the greater the risk of developing coronary heart disease.

While in hospital you may be seen by a dietitian and given information on a 'low fat' diet.

It is up to your doctor to decide if a 'low fat' diet is necessary after you go home. Your doctor may also start you on tablets prior to your discharge from hospital which will help lower your cholesterol.

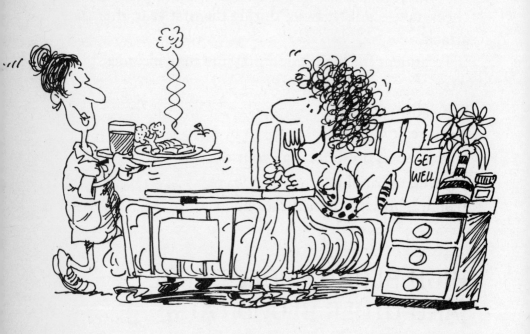

Triglycerides

Cholesterol and triglycerides together are known as lipids. These are commonly measured with a blood test.

If your blood triglyceride level is high you may need to reduce your alcohol and sugar intake. Remember that the narrowing of your coronary artery developed slowly over many years and will not suddenly become worse because you occasionally stray from your diet.

Australians would be much healthier if they consumed fewer foods that are high in animal fat (see the dietary advice on pages 55–9 for more information).

There are many 'low fat' diet books available at newsagents, bookshops and the National Heart Foundation of Australia.

OVERWEIGHT (OBESITY)

Many Australians are overweight.

Being overweight can cause high blood pressure and diabetes.

Extra weight does not, by itself, cause heart attack but after a heart attack it does become an undesirable burden for your heart.

Reducing the amount of fat in your diet, combined with regular moderate exercise, will go a long way towards helping you lose weight – remember fat has twice as many calories (kilojoules) as carbohydrate or protein (a teaspoon of butter is more than twice as fattening as a teaspoon of sugar).

Alcoholic drinks are also high in calories (kilojoules). Alcohol, in fact, has nearly twice as many calories as sugar.

You will lose weight after your heart attack if you follow a regular exercise programme and a healthy, balanced eating plan.

STRESS AND TENSION

There are many types of stress, for example:

Money troubles
Family worries
Work pressure
Inability to relax
Too much to do
Arguments
Driving in traffic

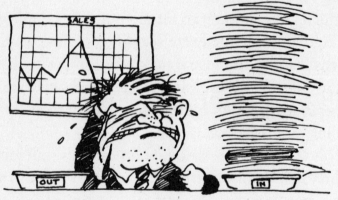

External Stresses

External stresses are things that happen to you which you find unpleasant and therefore stressful. For example, being caught in a traffic jam, the noise of construction work, or arguing constantly with a loved one. Some of these you may not be able to change but perhaps you can teach yourself to change your approach to them.

Others, such as arguing with a loved one, could possibly be changed. Discuss these stresses with your social worker and he or she will be able to advise you on how best to approach dealing with external stresses.

Internal Stresses

Internal stress is the stress that you place upon yourself. Do you expect too much of yourself and others around you? Do you worry a lot? Once again, you may have to learn to change your approach. Could you delegate some of your work to your colleagues to help relieve worry? Could you benefit by learning how to relax?

If you feel you need to learn how to relax discuss this with your doctor or the rehabilitation staff at your hospital. There are also a number of individuals and organisations offering courses in relaxation and meditation. Your local community centre will have information on relaxation.

LACK OF PROPER EXERCISE

In most people regular exercise tends to reduce the risk of future heart attacks and improves the efficiency of the heart muscle.

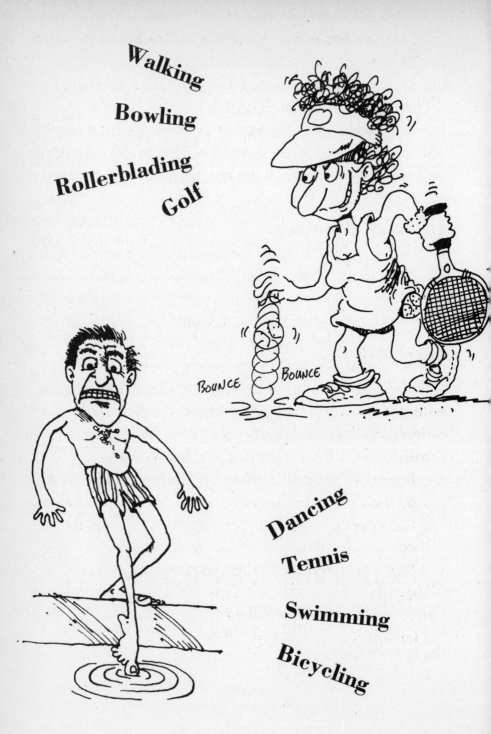

Walking

Bowling

Rollerblading   Golf

BOUNCE   BOUNCE

Dancing

Tennis

Swimming

Bicycling

Proper exercise means sustained effort for a period of 30 minutes 3 to 4 times a week rather than, for example, merely walking from the car park to work or sweeping the kitchen floor.

The average Australian settles down at about age 25 to a life of physical inactivity. Often when we do decide to exercise we tend to overdo it.

Don't overdo it, but work up gradually and regularly as you are instructed. Initially you should exercise under medical supervision. Most people who have had a heart attack will eventually return to a normal range of activities.

DIABETES

Diabetes (excess sugar in the blood) contributes to the development of atherosclerosis. If you are a diabetic it is therefore important to maintain good blood sugar control.

Diabetes is especially common in those who have a family history of this condition or who are overweight. If this applies to you or your family you should have a check-up for early detection of diabetes.

When a diabetic has a heart attack it is very important that in the first 2 weeks 'good control' is maintained. Insulin dosage may need frequent adjustment during this period.

HEREDITY

Even though you may inherit a tendency towards heart attack it is important to remember that prevention may be possible if you take steps to reduce the factors under your control.

Perhaps your family shares Risk Factors which can be corrected. Make sure you let your children know about the Risk Factors shared by your family.

A high proportion of teenagers in some communities already smoke, are overweight and have high blood cholesterol levels.

Why not use this opportunity to start your whole family on the path to healthier living?

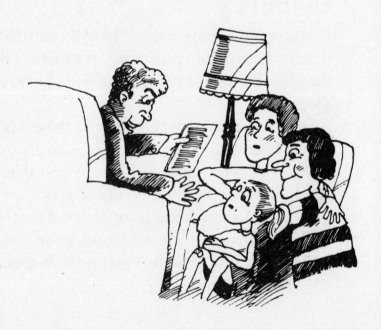

MENOPAUSE

The female hormone oestrogen has a cardioprotective effect; that is, it can protect women from heart disease. As this hormone decreases with menopause, women have an increased chance of developing heart disease.

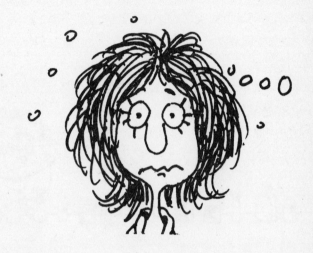

BEING MALE

As men are not protected by oestrogen they are at a higher risk of developing heart disease than women.

OVER 50 YEARS OLD

Natural wear and tear on the body increases the risk of developing heart disease.

MEDICATIONS

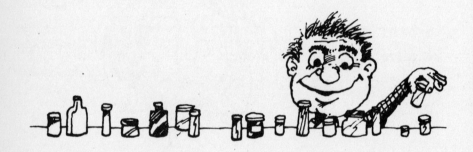

Some of you will be taking medications for different reasons and you should know:

- the name of the medication
- the dosage
- the reason why you are taking it.

Read medicine labels carefully.
Don't stop taking any medicine you have been prescribed without consulting your doctor first.

COMMONLY PRESCRIBED MEDICATIONS

Aspirin

Also known as Cardiprin, dispirin or Cartia, aspirin is commonly prescribed for heart attack patients as it helps thin the blood and assists preventing clot formation in the coronary arteries.

Nitrates

Nitrates are used in the treatment of angina because they help relax the coronary arteries allowing more blood to flow through. The names of some nitrates you might be prescribed are:

- Anginine (Glyceryl Trinitrate)
- Nitrolingual spray
- Isordil
- Imdur
- Nitroglycerin patches
- Nitrodisc
- Transiderm Nitro.

Beta Blockers

These are used in the treatment of angina, high blood pressure and abnormal heart rhythm. When used after a heart attack, or for angina, their main actions are to reduce the workload on the heart by slowing the heart rate, and to prevent disturbances of rhythm which may lessen the efficiency of the heart. Examples of beta blockers include:

- Atenolol (Tenormin or Noten)
- Metoprolol (Betaloc or Lopressor)
- Sotalol (Sotacor).

Calcium Antagonists

Calcium antagonists are used in the treatment of angina, high blood pressure and coronary artery spasm. The calcium antagonist Verapamil is also used to prevent disturbances of the heart rhythm. Examples of calcium antagonists include:

- Diltiazem (Cardizem)
- Amlodipine (Norvasc)
- Verapamil (Isoptin)
- Nifedipine (Adalat).

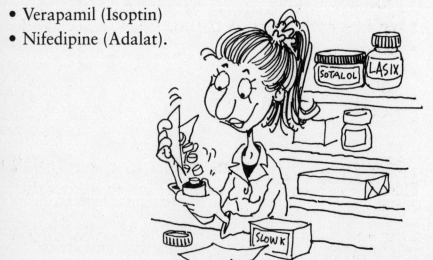

Ace Inhibitors

Ace inhibitors improve the heart's ability to pump and reduce blood pressure. Common ace inhibitors include:

• Captopril (Capoten)
• Enalapril (Renitec)
• Lisinopril (Zestril).

Diuretics

Diuretics prevent accumulation of water in the lungs and other parts of the body and are also used to treat high blood pressure. Some examples are:

• Lasix (Frusemide)
• Chlotride (Chlorothiazide).

Potassium

This is required by some people taking diuretics to replace potassium lost in the urine. Common examples include:

• Slow K (Potassium Chloride)
• Chlorvescent.

Hormone Replacement Therapy (HRT)

The use of hormone replacement therapy reduces the risk of heart attack and stroke in women after menopause. In addition, hormone replacement therapy can help lower cholesterol levels.

MEDICATION CHART

Name of medication	Date prescribed	When to take

Special instructions:

_____

_____

_____

_____

_____

GOING HOME

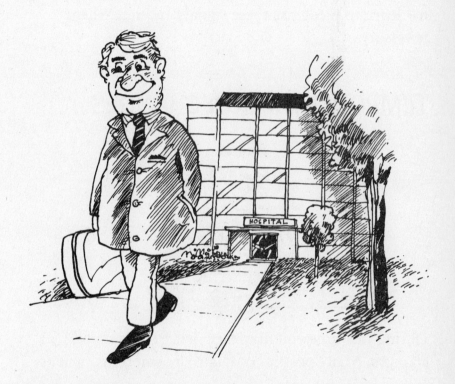

THE FIRST FEW DAYS AT HOME

It usually takes a few days to adjust to being home again (and no longer a patient!). This is tiring in itself and you should not expect to do much more than during your last days in hospital.

Don't be too impatient. There will be plenty of time for rapid improvement in the next few weeks.

We put restrictions on your activity at this time. You can easily become overtired (and possibly lose confidence in your ability to get well quickly) if you try to do too much too soon.

Your body will soon tell you when you are overdoing it – learn to recognise these signals and rest when necessary.

TEMPORARY MOOD CHANGES

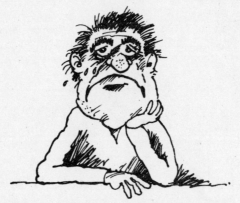

During this time you may experience some mood changes. Many people complain of symptoms such as:

- crying
- sleep difficulties
- irritability
- poor concentration and memory
- loss of interest

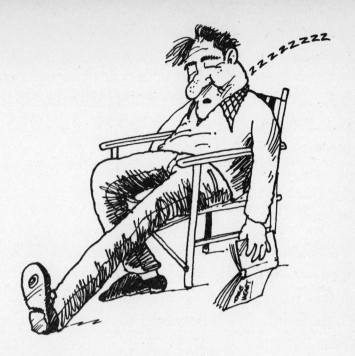

- tiredness
- emotions not usually experienced
- feelings of depression
- feelings of boredom.

These symptoms are common during the recovery period and usually disappear. However, if you still feel this way after a few weeks consult your doctor, social worker or cardiac rehabilitation clinic.

MYTHS

During this time well-meaning friends may tell you some myths which are not true.

Please don't take any notice of statements like these:

'You will never walk up stairs.'
'You will never have sexual intercourse.'
'You cannot lift your arms above your head.'
'You will never run again.'
'You will never be able to return to work.'
'You must not get excited.'
*'You may not do anything strenuous with your
left arm.'*
'You will never be able to do any lifting again.'

Another common myth is that you may not drink alcohol again. This is not true. You may drink alcohol in moderation.

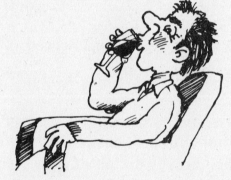

Excessive alcohol injures the heart muscle as well as other organs. However, unless you have been a heavy drinker in the past, you will do no harm by drinking 2 glasses of wine or beer per day.

People who are concerned for you may still tell you their own stories. You should be prepared for this so that you will find it easier to ignore them.

Here are some well-known stories that are best ignored:

'My neighbour had a heart attack and dropped dead after two weeks.'
'My neighbour died after his second heart attack.'

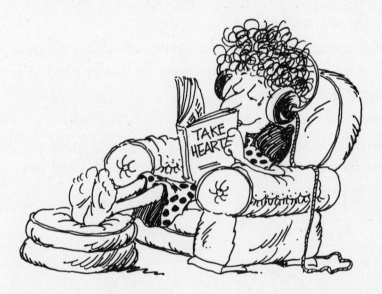

These days most patients recover completely from heart attacks and return to normal work and leisure activities within a few weeks.

WHAT YOU CAN DO

Most of the first week was spent in hospital so we shall talk about your first week at home as Week 2.

You may be unsure how much you can do in the first few weeks.

An individual plan will be worked out by the cardiac rehabilitation unit while you are in hospital, and we offer the following as guidelines only.

WEEK 2

- Get up and dressed.
- Walk around the house and garden at a leisurely pace.
- Make yourself a cup of tea – you no longer need to be waited on.
- Watch TV or read a book.
- Restrict your visitors – you may find them tiring in the first few days.
- Rest if you are tired.

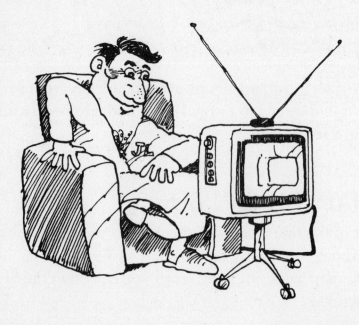

WEEK 3

By now you will be walking outside your house. Why not use your street light poles as a measurement – increase the distance that you walk by one light pole per day – and remember, you have to walk back again. Keep these things in mind before walking:

- Walk on level ground at a slow pace.
- Walking is best done in the morning.
- Try to schedule your walk so that you do not walk in the coldest part of the day in winter, or in the heat of the day in summer.

Other things you can do in this week include:

- Going out to dinner or to a relaxing movie.
- Being driven to visit your friends.
- Shopping with someone. (Don't carry the groceries at this stage.)
- Some light gardening.
- Light household duties. (Cooking a meal a day or washing dishes and cleaning up after meals.)
- Putting clothes in the washing machine. (But don't carry wet clothes out to the line.)

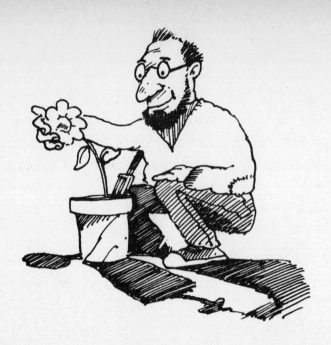

DON'TS DURING THE FIRST TWO WEEKS AT HOME (WEEKS 2 AND 3)

- Do not lift weights or do other straining exercises.
- Do not vacuum, sweep or do heavy cleaning.
- Do not wash the car.
- Do not drive the car.
- Do not rake leaves, or do heavy gardening.
- Do not swim, play tennis or golf.
- Do not mow the lawn.

WEEK 4

At this time the distance and pace of your walking will be increased progressively. Don't exercise for at least one hour following meals.

Wash the car – ready for when you start driving, as it is at about this stage that your doctor will suggest you resume driving your car.

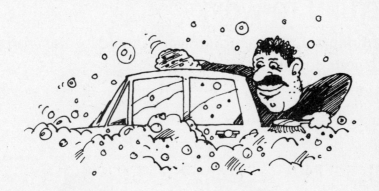

RESUMPTION OF SEXUAL ACTIVITY

Frequently, due to embarrassment, questions concerning sexual intercourse after a heart attack go unasked and unanswered.

However, at first you should avoid sexual intercourse in the following situations:

- for 2 to 3 hours after a heavy meal, excessive alcohol or exercise
- if you are very tired.

At first, techniques which require less physical exertion on your part could be tried. Whatever position was most comfortable before your heart attack may be the most appropriate.

If you are experiencing any difficulties please consult your doctor.

RETURN TO WORK

The timing of your return to work should be discussed with your doctor.

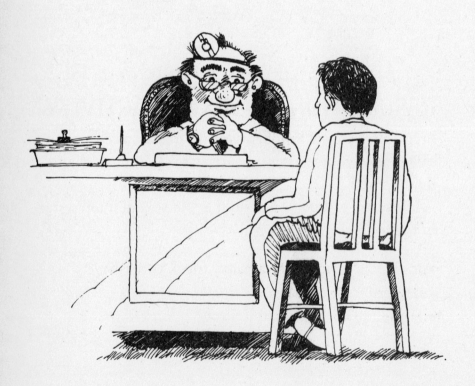

EXERCISING FOR FUTURE FITNESS

EXERCISING UNDER SUPERVISION

After you return home you may be invited to participate in a cardiac rehabilitation programme. The aim of the programme is to:

- assist you to achieve optimal psychological and social wellbeing through education and support for yourself and your family
- provide an exercise and educational programme to encourage cardiovascular fitness
- encourage you to adopt a lifestyle that limits the progression of atherosclerosis and minimises the risk of further cardiac events

- maximise physical, psychological and social recovery so that you can achieve a lifestyle that is as productive and personally satisfying as possible.

WALKING PROGRAMME

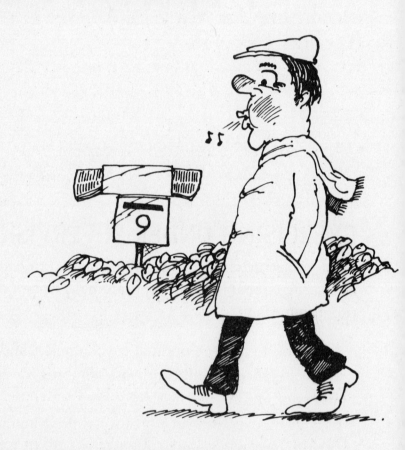

A walking programme is encouraged during rehabilitation. It is the simplest and most convenient exercise, and is a reliable method of improving your physical fitness.

Your walking distance and speed will be specified by the rehabilitation staff or by your doctor.

Rate of progress is very much an individual matter.

Conditions for Walking during Your Recovery Period

Some of these conditions have been mentioned earlier but they are repeated here to emphasise their importance.

- The ground should be relatively flat and level. Walking uphill greatly increases the work of the heart. If you cannot avoid climbing hills you should make sure you slow down. The same applies to walking into a head wind.
- Temperature extremes also increase the work of the heart. Try to time your walk so that you do not walk in the coldest part of the day in winter, or in the heat of the day in summer.
- Digestion makes additional demands on the heart. You should avoid vigorous exercise for an hour before and 2 hours after a meal.
- The heart often takes a few minutes to adjust to exercise. Always do some gentle warm-up exercises before you walk, or start your walk slowly.

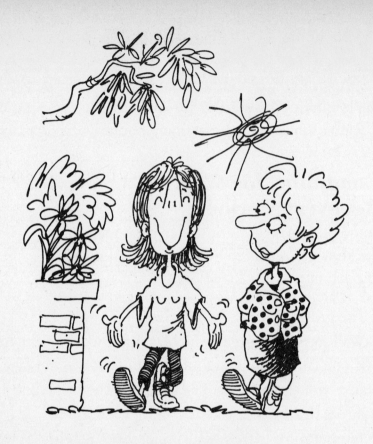

How Far Should You Walk?

The walking chart on page 52 is offered as a weekly guide. The amount of time spent walking depends on a number of factors, including your stage of recovery, age and previous physical fitness.

Check your distance and fitness category with your doctor before commencing this programme.

If you are unsure how much you should do, start with a shorter distance. The overall aim is to gradually increase your walking distance and to reduce the time it takes to walk this.

Do not be discouraged by periods of slower progress when it may seem you are not improving. This is common and is almost always temporary. If you experience this kind of set-back it may be best to drop back a stage until the walking becomes comfortable again.

Use the chart on page 52 to determine the amount of time you should spend walking while recovering from a heart attack. When you have fully recovered, walking should be maintained at a rhythmic, even pace for at least 30 minutes and should be performed at least 3 to 4 times per week.

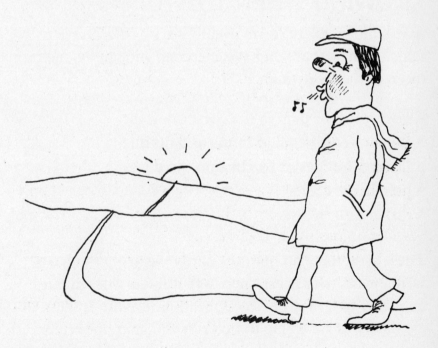

Graduated Walking Programme

Week	Distance
3	0.4 km (¼ mile)
4	0.8 km (½ mile)
5	1.2 km (¾ mile)
6	1.6 km (1 mile)
7	2.4 km (1½ miles)
8	3.2 km (2 miles)

KNOWING WHEN TO STOP

Safe limits of exercise are usually set by your body, which signals that you have exercised enough by one or more of the following:

- discomfort or pain in the chest or arms
- shortness of breath (panting and puffing)
- fatigue (feelings of exhaustion, tired legs)
- pain in the calves
- dizziness or nausea.

These symptoms do not necessarily mean anything is wrong with your heart, merely that it has worked hard enough and it may be necessary to reduce the amount of exercise you are trying to do. You will gain no further benefits by pushing beyond these 'barriers'.

Report any of the symptoms listed on the previous page to your doctor at your next visit.

EXERCISES TO AVOID DURING THE FIRST TWO MONTHS

There is one type of exertion which is not beneficial. This is exercise which involves 'straining'. Included in this category are:

• very heavy lifting and carrying
• pushing and pulling heavy objects, for example a car or refrigerator
• opening a stuck window.

If you have high blood pressure or angina it may be best to avoid these exercises.

THE FUTURE

Almost all people who recover from a heart attack are able to walk briskly, play golf, resume sex and engage in similar activities without trouble.

Now that you are on the way to recovery from this heart attack, take steps to reduce your chances of further trouble by modifying your lifestyle.

EXERCISE STRESS TEST

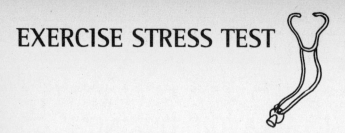

Many people are given an exercise stress test following their heart attack.

Your doctor may order this while you are an in-patient or some weeks after your heart attack.

This test records the heart beat during rest, exercise and immediate post exercise.

This simple procedure takes approximately 1 hour and is supervised by a doctor. The exercise may be achieved by riding a stationary bike or walking briskly on a treadmill.

During the test you are connected to an electrocardiograph machine so that changes in your heart are recorded. An electrocardiograph machine records the electrical impulses travelling through the heart muscle and can detect lack of blood supply to parts of the heart muscle.

You will be asked to fast for 4 hours before having the test.

You may need to cease some of your medications for 24 to 48 hours before this test. Your doctor will tell you if this is necessary.

Remember to wear comfortable clothes and sandshoes.

DIET AND HEART DISEASE

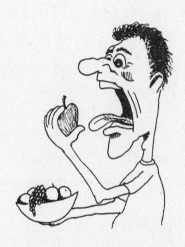

The foods we eat can influence blood vessel condition by affecting the build up of fatty deposits. Check with your dietitian and doctor what food is appropriate for you.

REDUCING YOUR RISK

The risk factors for heart disease that are influenced by diet are:

• high blood cholesterol

- excess weight
- high blood pressure.

By changing to a 'healthy diet' you can reduce your risk of heart disease.

HIGH BLOOD CHOLESTEROL

Cholesterol is a substance carried in the bloodstream. Some of it is made by the body itself and some comes from the food we eat. Blood cholesterol is required for normal living; however, when this level rises too high there is a risk of blood vessel damage and heart disease.

Your blood cholesterol level is affected much more by the amount of fat you eat than by the amount of cholesterol in your diet.

A high dietary fibre intake also assists with lowering cholesterol levels when combined with a low fat diet.

The recommended blood cholesterol level is less than 5.5 mmol/L.

LOWERING YOUR CHOLESTEROL

Reduce All Fat in Your Diet

All fats and oils are equally high in energy (kilojoules). Use fats sparingly and be watchful of hidden fats in foods, especially if you need to lose weight.

The type of fat you include in your diet is very important. As a general rule, saturated fats should be avoided completely and monounsaturated and polyunsaturated fats should be used sparingly.

Saturated Fats
Avoid saturated fats as they increase cholesterol.

These are found in meat fat, poultry skin, full-fat dairy products, cream, butter, cakes, pastries, coconut cream and fried foods, etc.

Monounsaturated Fats
Use these **sparingly**.

They are found in olive oil, canola oil, certain nuts and avocado.

Polyunsaturated Fats
Use these **sparingly**.

They are found in fish, polyunsaturated margarine, certain nuts and vegetable oils, for example, sunflower and safflower oil.

Both polyunsaturated and monounsaturated fat help lower cholesterol when eaten in small amounts.

Cholesterol in Foods
The amount of cholesterol in foods is less important than the fat content. Advertised 'low cholesterol' foods are not necessarily low fat, so read food labels carefully.

ENJOYING A HIGH FIBRE DIET

Soluble Fibre

Soluble fibre will assist in lowering cholesterol and is found in oats, rice and barley bran, legumes and pulses.

Insoluble Fibre

Insoluble fibre helps to fill you up and promote bowel regularity and is found in wholemeal breads and pastas, wholegrain breakfast cereals, wholewheat flour, brown rice, fruit and vegetables.

HELPFUL HINTS FOR A HEALTHY DIET

Attain and maintain a 'healthy weight' by:

- including regular exercise in your daily routine
- reducing the total amount of high fat foods eaten in the diet
- cooking food in ways that do not require adding fats and oils, for example, steaming, microwaving, barbequing, stewing, grilling and marinading
- trimming all visible fat from meats and skin from chicken **before** cooking
- using low/reduced fat dairy products, that is, milk, cheese and yoghurt

- using 'monounsaturated oils' **sparingly** in cooking, for example, canola and olive oil
- increasing the amount of high fibre foods eaten in the diet by filling up on foods that are of plant origin, for example, wholegrain bread and cereals, fruit and vegetables, grains and pasta
- drinking alcohol in moderation (recommended no more than 2 glasses per day)
- decreasing the amount of salt used in cooking and added at the table, and by using reduced salt products where possible.

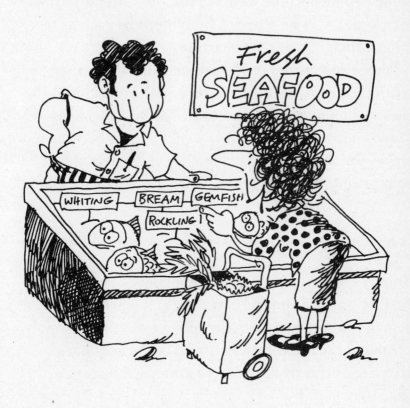

ANGINA

PAINS!

Some people become 'heart-conscious' after a heart attack and may be worried by symptoms such as fatigue, palpitations, or heartburn.

People sometimes have various pains when they return home. Most of these arise in the muscles of the chest wall and are unimportant. Pains of this kind usually subside within a few weeks as you become more active. Some people do experience chest discomfort or pain arising from the heart. This pain is called 'angina'.

WHAT IS ANGINA?

Angina is the heart muscle's complaint of poor circulation – it is not a heart attack. It is when the heart's demand for oxygen from the blood exceeds the supply.

Angina is caused by narrowing of the coronary arteries. This is usually due to atherosclerosis (see page 9).

Angina may also be caused by coronary artery spasm. Spasm is the involuntary contraction of the coronary artery that causes a temporary narrowing of the artery.

A number of factors may hasten the narrowing of coronary arteries. These are the same Risk Factors that increase your chances of having a heart attack (see page 20).

Remember! Reducing your Risk Factors reduces angina.

Angina is not usually severe and often disappears with rest. It can also be greatly relieved with medications that improve blood flow to the heart muscle and relieve discomfort within 3 to 5 minutes.

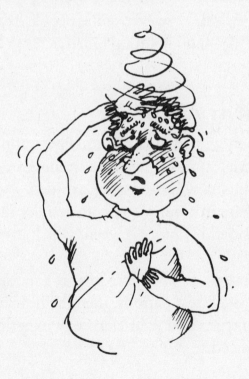

RECOGNISING ANGINA

Angina is not felt the same way by everyone. The feeling can be any of the following:

- pain or tightness in the centre of the chest
- pain or tightness in one or both arms
- pain in the throat or jaw
- a feeling of discomfort or pressure in the chest.

Angina is the signal that a part of the heart muscle is temporarily not receiving enough oxygen. This occurs when your heart muscle is working a little harder than usual due to excitement, exercise, walking quickly or eating a large meal. However, some people experience angina while sleeping or sitting quietly.

MANAGING ANGINA

While a person with angina can usually continue a normal lifestyle, some of the more strenuous activities that induce angina will need to be avoided.

When you are in a hurry to do an activity the heart requires considerably more oxygen, which in turn may lead to angina.

If you choose to do your activities at a moderate pace, allowing for short rest periods, then the heart will require less oxygen and your chance of experiencing angina is reduced.

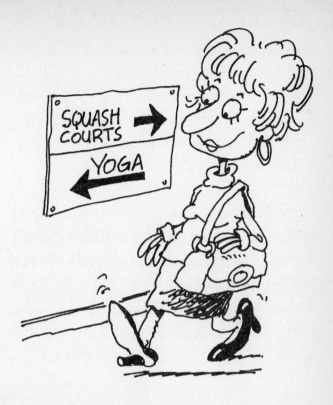

Notice your usual pattern of angina and be alert to any changes. Notify your doctor if:

- pain persists
- pain becomes more frequent
- pain is brought on with very little exertion.

Despite medications and activity adjustments your doctor may recommend an exercise stress test (see page 54) and/or coronary angiography (see page 68) in order to evaluate the location and extent of the atherosclerosis in the coronary arteries.

MEDICATION FOR ANGINA

If you experience angina you will need to know how to take your prescribed medication. Either Anginine tablets or Nitrolingual spray will be prescribed.

Anginine tablets and Nitrolingual spray are not harmful nor addictive.

Remember the following:

- Keep your medication with you at all times.
- Keep Anginine tablets in their original bottle and make sure the lid fits tightly as the tablets deteriorate when exposed to light. You may like to ask your chemist about a pharmacy-approved container for better protection against light exposure.

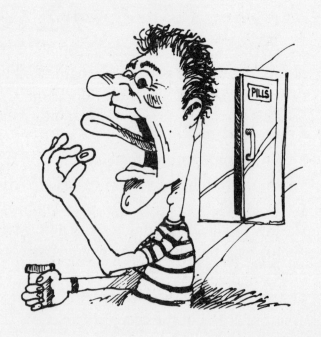

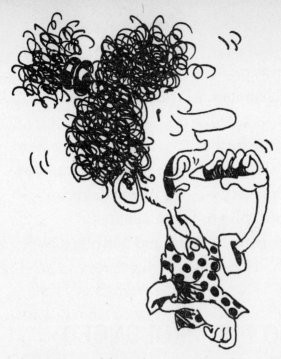

- Anginine tablets deteriorate after a period of time.
  Write the date on the tablets when you buy them.
  They last only 6 months when unopened. Write the
  date on the bottle when you open it. Once the bottle
  is opened the tablets will last only 3 months.
  Nitrolingual spray lasts for up to 2 years. Make sure
  you check the expiry date on your spray.
- Place the tablet or the spray under the tongue. Allow
  the tablet to dissolve or chew it until dissolved in your
  mouth. Do not swallow it. After spraying it is best to
  close your mouth so that you receive the full benefit
  of the Nitrolingual.

- Until you know your reaction to your angina medication it is advisable to sit or lie down for at least 10 minutes after using it, as you may experience dizziness from a temporary lowering of blood pressure.
- Anginine may cause headaches. If these occur, a ¼ or ½ tablet may be sufficient to relieve chest discomfort.
- Angina medication may be used before doing an activity you know will produce angina.
- Discard all old Anginine tablets and Nitrolingual spray.

WHAT TO DO FOR PROLONGED ANGINA PAIN

If pain is unrelieved 5 minutes after taking 1 tablet or 2 sprays, take a second tablet or spray a third or fourth time. If severe pain persists over the next 5 minutes take a third tablet. It is recommended you do not take more than 4 sprays because the spray is absorbed much faster than the tablets. If severe pain persists for more than 20 minutes after onset, seek help by ringing the Australia-wide emergency number:

- Dial 000
- Ask for MICA (Mobile Intensive Care Ambulance).

CORONARY
PROCEDURES

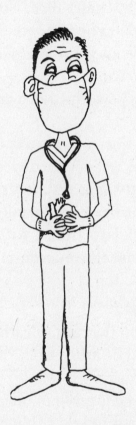

Coronary angiography, coronary angioplasty, the insertion of a coronary stent and cardiac surgery are common investigative and interventional procedures. This chapter offers a detailed description of those procedures.

CORONARY ANGIOGRAPHY

After you recover from a heart attack your doctor may recommend you undergo the procedure known as 'coronary angiography'. The coronary angiography may be performed during your stay in hospital or as an elective procedure at a later time. Coronary angiography is an X-ray procedure that is used to examine the arteries of your heart with a special camera.

The procedure is performed in a catheterisation laboratory.

The test enables doctors to detect the presence of any coronary disease in arteries narrowed or blocked by atherosclerosis (fatty deposits). It also assesses how well the chambers of the heart are functioning. The total procedure generally lasts from 1 to 2 hours and you will be awake throughout the procedure.

The Procedure

When transferred to the cardiac catheterisation laboratory you will be asked to lie on a narrow bed under an X-ray camera.

A local anaesthetic is given in the groin or elbow crease and the doctor inserts a thin plastic tube (catheter) into an artery in either the groin or elbow and threads it into the section of the aorta (main artery in the body) from where the coronary arteries originate. This procedure is completely painless.

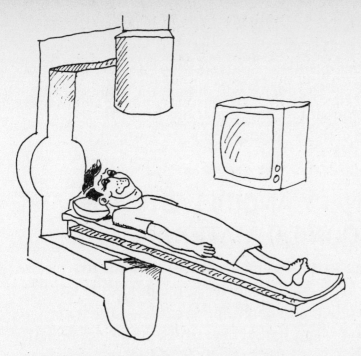

A dye is then injected through the tubing into the coronary arteries and the heart chambers. Pictures are taken and recorded on videotape and cine film. The doctor gives several injections of dye while taking X-ray photographs, moving the bed so that the vessels can be viewed from several angles. (You are secured to the bed.)

You may feel a sensation of warmth, flushing or tingling when the dye is injected but the sensation lasts only 20 to 30 seconds.

Once the procedure is finished the catheter is removed and a pressure bandage or pressure device is applied over the area of insertion to prevent bleeding.

On returning to the ward you will be asked to rest keeping your leg or arm straight. It is also necessary for you to drink plenty of fluids so as to flush the dye from your system. The doctor will discuss the results of the investigation and recommendations for further treatment with you before you leave hospital.

CORONARY ANGIOPLASTY (BALLOON DILATATION)

This is a procedure using a similar technique to coronary angiography. However, the procedure is different in that a balloon-tipped cardiac catheter is inflated to try and flatten the fatty deposits (atheroma) against the artery wall and enlarge the passageway for increased blood flow.

This technique may be recommended by your doctor as an alternative form of treatment to coronary artery bypass surgery.

Patient selection for this treatment is dependent on the number of arteries narrowed and the severity of the coronary artery disease.

All patients will have previously undergone coronary angiography. The decision for 'balloon dilatation' is discussed with you by the specialist who performs this procedure.

The procedure carries with it a small risk of surgical intervention. It is therefore normal practice to have a cardiac surgeon and theatre facilities available during the 'balloon' treatment.

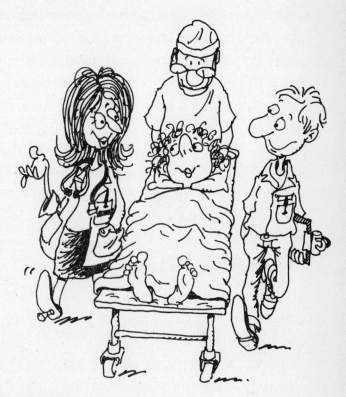

The Procedure

The hospital stay is usually about 1 day.

You will be asked to fast for 4 hours prior to the procedure and your groin will be shaved.

On transfer to the catheter laboratory a local anaesthetic is given in the groin and a narrow catheter with a balloon tip is passed into a blood vessel and advanced to the narrowed coronary artery requiring dilatation.

The balloon-tipped catheter is then inflated to stretch the wall of the artery at the site that is narrowed.

The procedure takes approximately 2 hours.

To minimise the small risk of bleeding post procedure a small tube is left in the groin for a few hours. When the tube is removed a pressure bandage is applied.

You will be required to remain resting in bed keeping the leg straight for 4 hours following removal of the tube from the groin.

The specialist will discuss the results of the procedure with you as soon as he or she has reviewed the X-ray films taken during the procedure.

CORONARY STENT

A stent is a small metal-coiled device used to provide structural support to a vessel in order to keep the artery open. A coronary stent is implanted following coronary angioplasty. If you are to receive a coronary stent, your doctor may ask you to follow certain instructions. For several days prior to the procedure you will be asked to take aspirin and other prescribed medications. You will need to let your doctor know if you:

• cannot take aspirin
• are taking any medications
• have any history of drug allergies
• have a history of bleeding problems.

CARDIAC SURGERY

Sometimes following coronary angiography your doctor may recommend coronary artery bypass surgery.

This surgery uses a vein or artery from the leg or from behind the breastbone to increase the supply of blood to the heart by bypassing an obstruction in one or more arteries.

One end of the vein graft is sewn into the aorta above the original opening to the coronary artery. The other end is attached to the coronary artery below the obstruction. That is why the operation is called a coronary artery bypass graft.

Immediately after the operation you will spend 12 to 24 hours in the Intensive Care Unit. The remainder of your hospital stay (about 5 to 7 days) will be spent in a cardiac surgical ward.

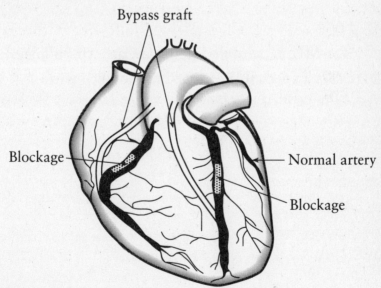

Diagram showing coronary artery bypass grafts after cardiac surgery

Community Information

Anyone, anywhere may suddenly be faced with an emergency such as drowning or sudden collapse; therefore, it is very important for everyone to know how to give basic life support (i.e. cardiopulmonary resuscitation).

Organisations that teach this are:

- St Johns Ambulance
- National Heart Foundation
- State Ambulance Service
- Red Cross.

If you think someone is having a heart attack:

- Dial 000
- Ask for MICA (Mobile Intensive Care Ambulance). MICA is a specially equipped ambulance with specially trained officers.

Glossary

Angina   Pain caused by lack of oxygenated blood supplied to the heart as a result of coronary artery disease.

Anginine   A rapidly acting tablet used for chest pain by being placed under the tongue.

Anterior descending artery   Artery supplying the front of the heart.

Aorta   Major blood vessel leaving the heart that supplies the entire body with oxygenated blood.

Artery   Blood-carrying vessel.

Atheroma   Another name for 'atherosclerosis'.

Atherosclerosis   Also known as 'coronary artery disease', this is the fatty build-up of plaque that causes heart disease.

Balloon dilatation   see Coronary angioplasty.

Cardiac   Relating to the heart.

Cardiac surgery   Surgery of the heart and its arteries.

Cardiopulmonary resuscitation   Attempting to revive someone from apparent death and/or unconsciousness.

Cardiovascular   Pertaining to the heart and its vessels.

Catheter   A flexible or rigid hollow tube.

Catheter laboratory   A room where procedures are performed under X-ray.

Cholesterol   A normal constituent of blood which is produced by our bodies and is also found in many of the foods we eat. An excessive blood cholesterol level (more than 5.5 mmol/L) can increase the risk of heart disease.

Cine film   A type of film that can record X-ray images.

Circumflex coronary artery   Artery that supplies the lateral surface of the heart.

Collaterals   Vessels that can develop when your existing vessels become diseased.

Coronary   Relating to the arteries that supply the heart tissue.

Coronary angiography   An X-ray procedure whereby dye is injected to examine the arteries of the heart (coronary arteries).

Coronary angioplasty   An X-ray procedure where a balloon-tipped catheter is inserted into the narrowed coronary artery. The small balloon is inflated and deflated for several seconds to try to flatten the build up (atherosclerosis) against the artery wall. This improves blood flow to the heart muscle.

Coronary artery bypass surgery   Surgery to the heart's arteries to bypass blockages.

Coronary occlusion   A complete blockage of the coronary artery.

Coronary stent   A metal coiled device which is inserted into the coronary artery to keep it open. A coronary stent is implanted following a coronary angioplasty.

Coronary thrombosis   A clot within the coronary artery.

Diabetes   A disease in which the body's ability to use sugar is impaired.

Echocardiograph   An ultrasound examination of the heart that records the movement of the heart valves and chamber walls.

Electrocardiograph (ECG)   A test that records the electrical impulses travelling through the heart muscle. The ECG is often helpful in detecting abnormal heart beats and areas of heart muscle damage or lack of blood supply.

Enzymes   Complex proteins that are produced by the body's cells and can be detected in the bloodstream after a heart attack.

Exercise stress test   A special test to measure the heart's function under stress.

GTN   (Glyceryl Trinitrate) An intravenous form of Anginine.

Heparin   An intravenous medication that causes thinning of the blood.

Heredity   The genetic characteristics transmitted from one's parents.

Hypertension   Elevation of the blood pressure.

Insoluble fibre   Fibre that is incapable of being dissolved and therefore aids digestion.

Intensive care unit   A highly specialised area where a patient is closely monitored.

Lipids   Fatty acids produced by the body. They are a normal constituent of blood just like cholesterol.

Menopause   A period of irregular menstruation prior to complete cessation of menstruation occurring in women usually between the ages of 45 and 50.

MICA   A highly equipped intensive care ambulance with officers specially trained to deal with all types of emergencies.

mmol/L   A measurement relating to blood chemistry.

Monounsaturated fat   A type of fat found in olive or canola oil; lower in cholesterol than saturated fats.

Myocardial infarction   The medical term for 'heart attack'.

Nitrolingual spray   A rapidly acting spray used for chest pain by being sprayed under the tongue. (An alternative to the Anginine tablet.)

Pericarditis   A short-term problem caused by inflammation of the 'pericardium' which may occur after a heart attack, but generally disappears after a few days.

Pericardium   The sac that encloses the heart.

Polyunsaturated fat   A type of fat found in margarines and cooking oils; lower in cholesterol than saturated fats.

Pulmonary artery   Artery that carries blood to the lungs to be oxygenated.

Right coronary artery   Artery that supplies the right

side and base of the heart.

Saturated fat   An animal fat found in meat and dairy products; very high in cholesterol.

Thrombolytic therapy   Intravenous Streptokinase and TPA are two of the 'clot dissolving' medications that can be given to abort or decrease the size of a heart attack through the procedure known as 'thrombolytic therapy'.

Triglycerides   Another important blood fat and source of energy. If your triglyceride levels are high (more than 2 mmol/L) you may need to reduce your sugar and alcohol intake. High levels increase the risk of heart disease.

✂ **Reader Response Survey**

We hope this booklet has been helpful. We invite your suggestions for any improvements to be made to subsequent editions.

We would be grateful if you would complete this page and return it to:

Take Heart
Viking
c/- Penguin Books Australia Ltd
487 Maroondah Highway
Ringwood Vic. 3134

Where did you obtain your copy? _____
_____
How many copies did you obtain? _____
Was the price acceptable?_____
Was it easy to understand?_____
If not, which areas were unclear? _____
_____
_____
_____

What were the main advantages you gained from reading this book?_____
_____
_____
_____

Any other comments?_____
_____
_____
_____

Notes

Notes